The Prepper's Guide To Ebola Survival

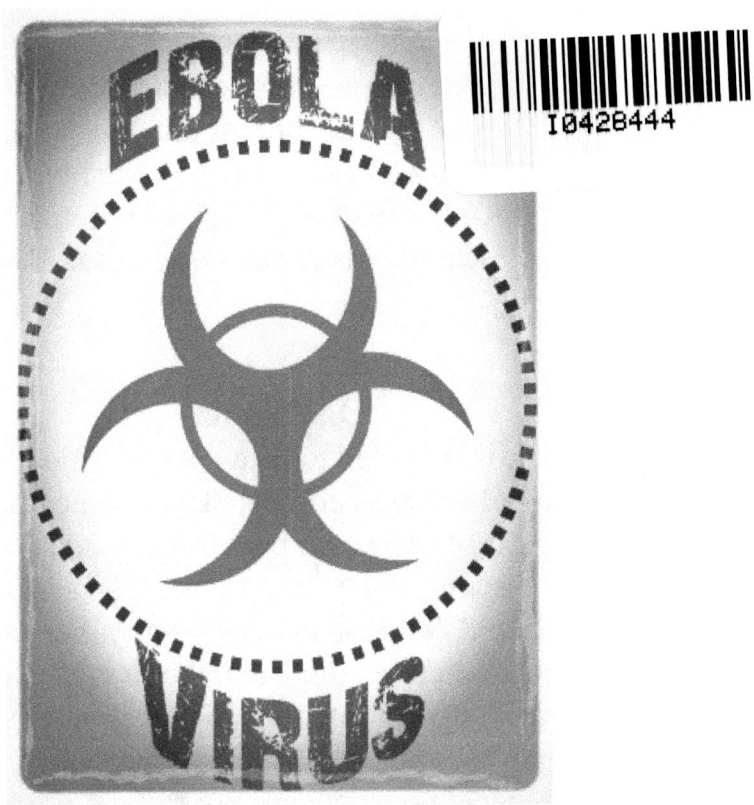

How to Identify, Prevent, And Survive A Possible Global Outbreak

By Ron Johnson

Disclaimer

This book is intended to be a general guide, to raise
awareness, and to help people make informed decisions in
the context of their own personal circumstance. As
everybody's circumstances are different, so are the remedies
you should seek. While many of the recommendations in this
book can be applied by almost anybody regardless of their
conditions they are not intended to and should not be relied
upon to replace personal medical advice.
The author accepts no responsibility for any loss or injury, be
it personal or financial, as a result for the use or misuse of
the information in this book. If you have any doubts or
concerns after reading this book, please speak to a doctor or
other qualified person before taking any actions.

Contents

Introduction

Chapter 1
What Is Ebola, How Can It Be Contracted And What Are The Symptoms?

Chapter 2
What Is The Possibility Of Ebola Becoming A Global Pandemic?

Chapter 3
How Is Ebola Diagnosed?

Chapter 4
Steps To Prevent Contracting Ebola

Chapter 5
What to Do If Someone You Know Becomes Infected

Introduction

With all the media outlets reporting new stories every day concerning new cases of the Ebola virus, it is imperative for everyone to learn more about it. You may be asking, what causes the Ebola virus? What are the symptoms? What can you do to avoid contracting it? Finally, what to do if you suspect you have it?

This book answers all of these questions, and some you haven't yet thought to ask. It is meant to enlighten the whole world on the threats that Ebola is posing to the entire world. It also highlights the actions that the nation of the world are taking to fight against this deadly disease.

Chapter one describes what Ebola is and how you can contract the virus. It also gives great details about the signs and symptoms.

Chapter two elaborates on how Ebola has become a global threat and explained the actions that the entire world are taking in the fight against this global pandemic.

In the third chapter, it highlights the steps that you must take once diagnosed, while chapter four provides the measures that are being taken to help stop the contraction and spread of Ebola.

Chapter five, six and seven shows the steps that you should take in the case you contract the Ebola virus. It also explains what you should not do once you discover that you have a deadly disease.

Chapter 1

What Is Ebola, How Can It Be Contracted And What Are The Symptoms?

Ebola is an infectious disease, which spreads by the way of contact with infected bodily fluids. Its cause is the Ebola virus or Filovirus. The Ebola virus (EVD), formerly known as Ebola hemorrhagic fever, causes an acute illness in humans, often fatal if left untreated. Animals act as initial carriers, and then the virus begins to spread via human-to-human transmission.

Ebola affects not only human beings, but also some mammals, and its symptoms typically start from two days to 2-3 weeks after contraction. Sore throat, fever and muscle pain are signs of the disease. Vomiting, rashes and diarrhea are also common; the liver and kidneys diminish their function. At this point, internal and external bleeding occur. Six to sixteen days after the appearance of the symptoms, the infected may die due to fluid loss.

The Ebola virus was first discovered in Sudan and The Democratic Republic of Congo (DRC). Its outbreak in the region of Sudan claimed the lives of 284 people with a mortality rate of 53 percent. The virus emerged a few months after in DRC and was referred to as the Ebola-Zaire (EBOZ). In this period, the region experienced the highest rates in mortality whereby the death toll climbed to more than 300 people. Researchers from across the world combined their efforts to fight the disease – this, however did not result in the prevention of the disease. To this day, a proven remedy for the Ebola disease (one that researchers have tested and were available for human use) has not been developed.

To achieve a better understanding of the current Ebola outbreak and its implications, we should return to the disease's historical background. The Ebola virus disease first appeared in two simultaneous outbreaks in 1976 in remote villages in Sudan and the Democratic Republic of Congo. The latter case occurred in a settlement near the Ebola River, from which the virus derives its name.

There was another outbreak of Ebola in 1989, known as Ebola Reston (EBOR). In this case, the virus was found in monkeys imported from Reston, Virginia and Mindanao in the Philippines.

Now, the Ebola virus has emerged again in West Africa - Liberia, Sierre Leone, Nigeria and other surrounding countries (first cases notified in March 2014). The mortality rate of this outbreak is the highest since the virus' discovery in 1989, thousands of lives being lost each day. It is the largest, most elaborate Ebola outbreak since the discovery of the virus back in 1976. There have been more deaths and cases of infection in this outbreak than in all the other combined. It started in Guinea, spreading across land borders to Liberia and Sierra Leone, by land to Senegal, and by air to Nigeria.

Countries with weak health systems are affected most severely – Guinea and Liberia, among others. They lack the infrastructural and human resources to handle the outbreaks, having only recently emerged from prolonged periods of instability.

The average Ebola virus case fatality rate is around 50%. Death rates have varied from 25% to 90% in past outbreaks. What makes the present outbreak a serious problem on an international level is the fact that the virus is spreading in highly populated urban areas. In previous cases of Ebola outbreaks that happened in relatively isolated rural areas, where people travel less, has made the disease outbreak not able to grow into a full-blown epidemic.

The contraction of Ebola

The Ebola virus can be contracted easily by touching the bodily fluids of an infected animal or person. As far as we know, the virus being airborne is not possible in the natural environment. Fruit bats are the regular carriers of Ebola in nature - that means; they can spread the virus without being affected themselves.

Humans are mostly infected through contact with dead and living animals that have been infected by the bats. After humans contract it, the disease begins to spread between people as well. Ebola can be transmitted by male survivors through their semen for a period of two months. In diagnosing EVD, diseases with similar symptoms are first eliminated. These diseases are cholera, malaria and viral hemorrhagic fevers. Initially, health workers test the blood samples for viral RNA, EBD and viral antibodies, so they are sure to make an accurate diagnose of the patient's condition.

Coordinated series of medical services are essential in order to control the outbreak. A particular level of community engagement is also a must. Contact tracing and detection should be done very rapidly, followed by quick access to specific laboratory services. The speed at which the infected attain access to laboratory services matters a lot. The infected need to be properly managed. Also, people in the community should dispose of the deceased properly – either through burial or cremation. The process of preventing the disease includes reducing the spread of the disease from infected humans, although one should keep in mind infected animals are also a problem. Bush meat (wild game meat, often sold in local markets) is also a potential source of infection. People, handling it should wear protective clothing. As an additional measure, the bush meat should be cooked thoroughly before consumption.

In any case, people should wash their hands and wear proper clothing when they are dealing with infected individuals or animals. You should handle all samples of body tissues and fluids with a lot of care.

Causes

The source of the Ebola virus is non-human primates in Africa, which includes monkeys and chimps. Medical research in the Philippines discovered a milder strain of Ebola in pigs and monkeys. Scientists found out that the Marburg virus also exists in monkeys, fruit bats, and chimps.

Transmission process from animals to humans

Medical researchers believe that infected animals transmit these two viruses to humans though their body fluids. A list of the common fluids follows:

- **Waste Products:** The Marburg virus has infected a number of mine workers and visitors. The workers contract the virus in their workplace by touching infected bats' excrements. Tourists who visit the caves also get infected in the same way.
- **Blood:** The spread of the virus accelerates when people consume already infected animals. Several researchers have also contracted the disease.

Person-to-person Transmission

Infected people become contagious after developing the symptoms. Family members are most vulnerable because they get infected while taking care of the sick relatives or preparing their dead relatives for burial.

All medical personnel dealing with infected people must use protective gear such as gloves and surgical masks. Reports show that numerous medical centers in West Africa reuse syringes and needles. It explains why this region has experienced some of the worst outbreaks of Ebola. The epidemic grows when local health workers use contaminated equipment.

The symptoms of Ebola

The Ebola virus has various symptoms, which this chapter will highlight. The disease has a short incubation period (incubation is the time interval from the infection to the start of the symptoms, ranging from 2 to 21 days). Keep in mind that humans become infectious after developing the

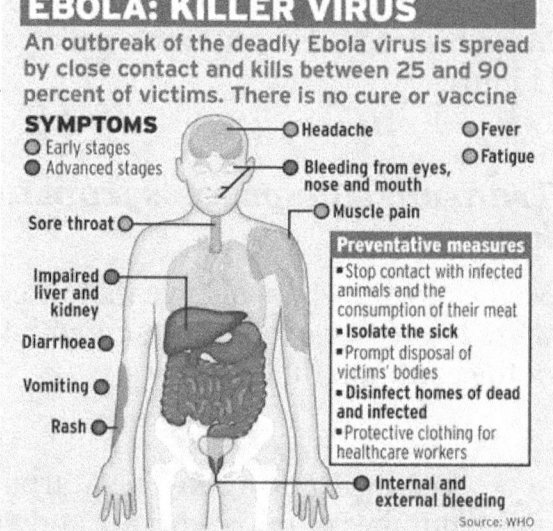

symptoms. The initial signs are muscle fatigue, sudden fever, headache, muscle pain and sore throat. The second stage involves diarrhea, vomiting, impaired liver and kidney function, rashes and, afterwards, often occurs internal and external bleeding. The blood oozes from the gums and stool. Various laboratory tests have indicated low platelet, white and red blood cells count, as well as increased liver enzymes.

The Ebola symptoms start appearing in between 2 to 21 days after making contact with infected people or animals. Usually, the signs of infection appear between the eight and tenth day.

Superior supportive clinical care is necessary for patients to recover from Ebola. People who recover from Ebola develop antibodies, which can sometimes last over ten years.

Chapter 2

What Is The Possibility Of Ebola Becoming A Global Pandemic?

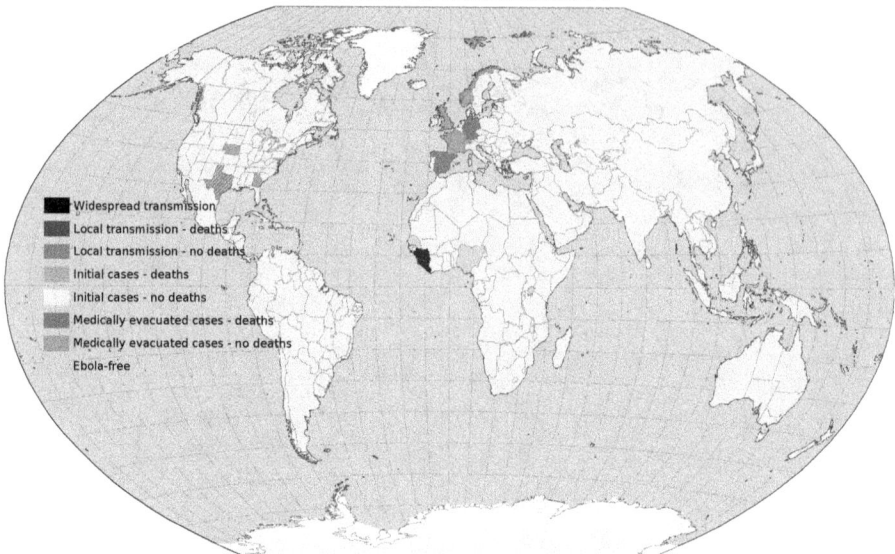

Above image shows the places effected by Ebola as of 1st October 2014

There are many reasons why Ebola might be a global pandemic. First, we can say that Ebola is a very dangerous virus. In fact, Ebola has been identified as one of the most infectious diseases on earth. The biggest problem is that the Ebola disease has one of the highest mortality rates. The case becomes clearer when we compare it to other diseases. To do that, we would have to consider various factors: the speed at which death occurs and the shock, associated with secondary infections. Currently, the disease has a fatality rate of 50%, which is very high compared to other fatal, infectious diseases.

Ebola - a global menace?

Various world leaders consider Ebola to be a significant

threat. The most recent, brutal outbreak is raging in several West African countries and is the largest, most complex outbreak of the virus ever recorded. The death toll of the Ebola outbreak has risen to 4,000. Additional cases of the disease have occurred in Spain as well as the United States. It clearly shows that the Ebola disease is now a global threat. Health organizations around the world have drawn up a number of predictions of the impact the virus will have on the world by 2015. The Center for Disease Control (CDC), based in the US, has also done thorough research on the subject. The Ebola threat will have claimed 550,000 people by January 2015, according to them.

Chapter 3

How Is Ebola Diagnosed?

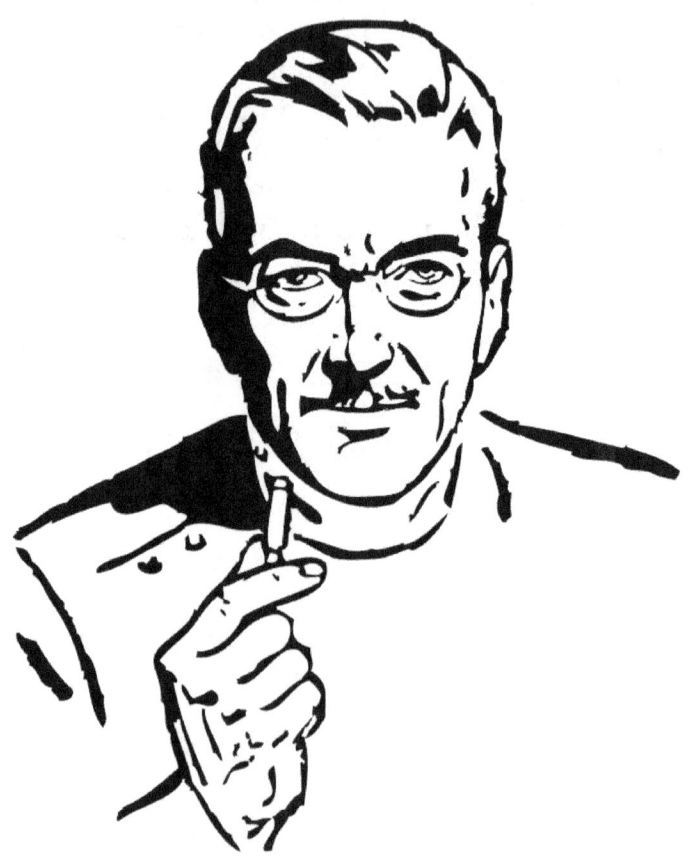

Distinguishing between Ebola and other diseases with similar symptoms - malaria, meningitis and typhoid fever is not easy to do. It is mostly because all of them are infectious. You can confirm medically that you are dealing with the Ebola virus by following these steps:

- The enzyme-linked immune-sorbent assay is an antibody-capture;

- Health workers perform detection tests on the

antigen capture;

- Test on serum naturalization;
- Electron microscopy;
- Healthcare professionals use cell structure for virus isolation;
- The reverse transcriptase polymerase which is a chain reaction assay is carried out.

Researchers should note that samples from patients are extremely dangerous. They constitute a serious biohazard. Therefore, when laboratory tests are carried out, all maximum biological safety precautions should be taken.

Diagnosis and Tests

Ebola, as well as Marburg hemorrhagic fever, has some of the most severe symptoms to diagnosis. As indicated earlier, they have signs and symptoms very much alike to those of a number of different diseases.

Therefore, health workers might easily suspect that a person has Ebola - even when that is not the case. Doing a number of different blood tests will help to determine the cause for the infection.

Since aiming to prevent the growth of the epidemic, the CDC and other US-based healthcare institutions, are actively researching Ebola and developing various blood tests, intended to diagnose the illness more accurately. They have well-equipped laboratories, which they utilize to learn more about the Marburg, as well as Ebola virus.

Ebola is very difficult to diagnose in its earlier stages. It is simply because most of its symptoms are visible in patients suffering from other commonly occurring diseases. Health workers consider this one of the greatest issues in preventing further development of the epidemic.

To prevent the growth of the Ebola epidemic is key that local communities quarantine anyone, who has become infected. For instance, in Liberia, local people protested against the quarantine measures and rioted to free the isolated people. Apparently, this happened due to the lack of public knowledge about the disease and had grave results. Uninfected people should never come into contact with the blood or body fluids of Ebola-positive individuals. If you suspect that someone has contracted Ebola, you should immediately contact health professionals. They could collect samples and carry out various tests to reveal if a person has acquired the virus or not.

Below, we'll mention some of the laboratory tests, carried out on patients, in different stages of the disease's development. During the period immediately after the infection, the researchers should carry out various tests such as IgM ELISA, antigen-capture enzyme-linked immunosorbent assay testing and polymerase chain reaction (PCR).

In late stages of the disease's development or after the patient's recovery, healthcare workers carry out IgG and IgM antibodies tests. Health professionals do blood tests on deceased patients. Some of the tests conducted include Virus isolation, PCR and immunohistochemistry testing.

In what way can we improve the survival rate of Ebola patients? By treating the symptoms of the disease and rehydrating them. This process involves providing intravenous or oral fluids. In addition to that, the specific symptoms can also be treated. These steps are essential to improving the chances of survival, as - for now – no official remedy for the Ebola disease (EVD) exists. Despite the lack of an effective and proven treatment, there are several potential ways to heal infected individuals. These are immune therapies, drug therapies, and blood products. Currently, no licensed vaccines exist. However, researchers have singled out two of the potentially most effective vaccines for human safety testing.

Chapter 4

Steps To Prevent Contracting Ebola

Avoiding contact with the virus by all means is the perfect way to retain your health. In this chapter, we'll outline some measures that can prevent the disease from spreading:

- **Frequent hand-washing:** This is a common practice when dealing with infectious diseases. It is a crucial preventive measure that you should adopt. People need to wash their hands more frequently using soaped water or alcohol-based hand rubs, when the soap and water are not available. These need to contain at least 60% alcohol.

- **Avoiding outbreak areas:** you should inform yourself about current epidemics before travelling to foreign countries. Most up-to-date information is available on the Centers for Disease Control and Prevention website.

- **Do not Consume Bush Meat:** When visiting developing countries, it is important to avoid eating bush meat. It is the meat from wild animals. Some people consume meat from non-human primates, which local markets customarily offer.

- **Do not stay in contact with infected people:** All caregivers shouldn't make physical contact with body fluids and tissues of people suffering from Ebola. You should also avoid contact with semen, saliva and vaginal secretions. Keep in mind that people suffering from Ebola become most contagious when they reach the late stages of the virus' development.

- **Stick to the infection-control procedures:** All care-givers must wear protective clothing such as gloves, gowns, clothing, masks, as well as eye shields. The community has to quarantine anyone who might have contracted the disease. Furthermore, the needles need to be disposed of after use on Ebola patients. All other equipment has to undergo careful sterilization.

- **Avoid Handling Remains:** The bodies of people who have been affected by the Ebola or Marburg diseases are highly contagious. Groups of properly instructed people should be set up to bury the bodies. Everyone on these teams should use the appropriate safety equipment.

Chapter 5

What To Do If Someone You Know Becomes Infected?

If a person a friend or family member contracts Ebola, you should follow these guidelines to stay safe:

- Using a sanitizer to wash your hands regularly;
- On no account touch a patient's blood or bodily fluids;
- Do not handle objects that an Ebola patient has touched;
- Never touch the body of someone who has died of Ebola without protective clothing;
- Never touch bats as well as animals like apes because these are the common carriers of the Ebola virus;
- Do not visit hospitals where Ebola patients are being treated for the disease.
- If you feel any of the following signs of fever and any other symptoms such as diarrhea, vomiting, muscle pain, headache, bleeding and stomach pain, seek medical attention immediately.
- Do not travel if you suspect that you have acquired the Ebola virus.

What do in areas, where cases of Ebola are reported?

If you are travelling to countries that have cases of Ebola, you might need to heed this advice:

- You should never come close to anyone, who is infected with the virus;
- Never touch the body of a deceased Ebola patient;
- Never touch body fluids of infected people;
- Do not touch animals, in any case, because you might never know whether they are carriers of the Ebola virus.

How does Ebola spread?

The Ebola disease becomes highly contagious after the development of the symptoms. Consuming infected meat, coming into contact with infected objects or animals are common ways of contracting the Ebola. The transmission of the virus takes place via the fruit bats, which are the natural hosts of the Ebola virus. The first cases of Ebola among humans, involved people having close contact with bodily fluids of fruit bats and becoming infected. As a result, other types of wild animals were also carriers of the virus - monkeys, gorillas, porcupines and forest antelopes. However, unlike the fruit bats, the virus affects them. That is why, since the Ebola outbreak, people often find infected animals, dying or very ill.

Once the animal-to-human transmission has taken place, the virus proceeds to the next level where it can spread among humans. Those infected should not be allowed to share their personal effects with unaffected by the virus people.

Recently, many health workers have contracted Ebola. It happens while they are offering their medical services to patients and do not practice the biohazard safety precautions strictly.

During burial ceremonies, mourners must avoid coming in contact with the remains of those who died from the disease. People continue being infectious as long as their body fluids contain the deadly virus. For instance, male Ebola patients, having recovered from the illness, should avoid having sexual intercourse for seven weeks afterwards because their semen carries the infection from the disease.

How can I stay safe when I travel?

The HSE and various governments have also advised people to avoid making unnecessary travels to countries that have reported cases of Ebola. As of 2014, there are confirmed cases of Ebola in Sierra Leone, Liberia, and Guinea. Health workers report outbreaks of the disease in Nigeria and Senegal. Travelers from other countries can reduce the risk of being infected by avoiding crowded venues and events. Accordingly, attending funerals or visiting hospitals is not a good idea. However, travelers cannot be infected by handling money or groceries. Mosquito bites are also harmless when it comes to contracting Ebola.

Vaccine development

Many scientists worldwide are currently working on new vaccines. These are the drugs that will be able to protect people from the Ebola epidemic. The initial results are very promising. For now, researchers merely need to carry out further testing.

Apart from the development of vaccines, there is a lot we can do to counter the growth of the epidemic. People worldwide should be well informed about the ways in which the disease spreads. The Ebola virus can spread in numerous ways, the primary way being through direct contact with the patients. Contact with clothing, needles and bedding – any contaminated object - can also be a source of the disease.

If possible, avoid areas with cases of Ebola

- Avoid all areas, where Ebola cases have appeared. This year the disease has spread in several West and Central African countries. A key source of infection is hospital and healthcare facilities, due to lack of resources and infrastructure in countries where the outbreak is at its worst. Governments around the world are a vital source of updated information on affected areas. The Center for Disease Control is at the forefront of providing useful information about the disease.

- You should avoid, by all means, areas where health workers suspect cases of the disease to exist. If you visit those areas, make sure you avoid the healthcare services. However, if you suspect you are a carrier of the disease, then you would need to visit those facilities for treatment. Above all, never come into direct contact with Ebola patients.

- You should avoid everyone who has contracted the disease; direct contact will lead to becoming infected. Blood and other secretions are the sources of infection of Ebola.

- Avoid eating bush meat, as researchers believe that infected animals caused the first human cases of infection with the Ebola virus. The initial infection happened after people consumed the bush meat. If you chance to be in the area, where the Ebola disease is spreading, avoid buying, handling or eating wild game. It is critical for your safety.

Chapter 6

What To Do If You Suspect You May Have Ebola?

If you suspect having contracted Ebola, the first thing to do is to avoid travelling to other places. It is important, so you can make sure virus does not spread further. Then seek medical attention from the designated healthcare facilities.

When you receive your medical prescriptions, always follow the doctor's instructions and never skip taking your medication. Ebola needs thorough diagnosing, and this is impossible to achieve if you do not cooperate with the medical experts. Restricting yourself to a medical prescription might seem to be tedious but remember once you have contracted Ebola, it is a matter of life and death.

What not to do after contracting Ebola

Once you find out that you have contracted Ebola do not travel anywhere else. You should rather look for means and ways of reaching the medical facilities that are capable of handling your case. You should also try not to infect others because the Ebola virus can infect anyone near you quite quickly. Also consider doing the following:

Learn about the symptoms of the Ebola virus, so you be able to recognize it in its initial stages. When you are aware of the disease's signs, you can protect yourself from it more effectively. Keep in mind, healthcare professionals sometimes confuse these symptoms with those of other diseases – for example, malaria. The first symptoms start appearing around 48 hours after exposure, in rare cases only after a period of three weeks.

Typical symptoms of Ebola include fever, muscles aches, lack of appetite, vomiting, weakness, headaches and general weakness, rash and red eyes. Affected individuals also experience difficulties in swallowing and breathing. Below we'll outline some actions that you need to take after contracting Ebola:

Wear protective clothing

People who work in health facilities should wear protective clothing at all times to make sure they do not acquire the virus while handling Ebola cases. All volunteers and healthcare workers should follow these rules to the letter. The CDC recommends that all healthcare workers use disposable gowns, masks, goggles and wear at all times when they are around Ebola patients.

It is a must that you dispose safely of all clothing and bedding used to treat the infected people. Meanwhile, you should exercise extreme caution.

Always disinfect all medical equipment. It includes all items that come into contact with the victims. The sterilization has to be done immediately after use.

All medical equipment should be sterilized immediately and then rinsed. Allow the instruments to dry thoroughly; then pack them into a disinfectant pouch. Afterwards, you may label them appropriately. All the sterilization pouches should be placed upside down in the sterilization tray, so there is enough space in between them. In this way, steam can function properly as a sterilizing agent. You have to follow strictly the right procedures when operating the sterilizer. Finally, you can catalog the devices and label them as sterilized.

Always practice quarantine and barrier nursing for the infected patients

You should upkeep the highest level of security if you are dealing with infected people. Some hospitals have employed plastic zippers. These will help in reducing chances of getting in contact with sick people. In other hospitals, the patients are quarantined - that means, healthcare professionals separate them from the general public. When you take this precaution, chances of the disease spreading among healthy people are lowered.

If you are infected with Ebola

If you believe you have contracted the Ebola virus, you may be wondering, what should you do? The first step is to receive a diagnosis from a competent healthcare worker. Symptoms alone aren't enough to create a stable diagnose because they are often confused with symptoms of other diseases. If you suspect that the virus has affected you, go immediately to the nearest healthcare facility and ask that different blood tests are carried out on you.

Contact the CDC

CDC is the Center for Disease Control. You should report your case as soon as possible. When you reach out to the CDC, inform them about your illness and the area from which you are operating. It is imperative to keep the disease contained at all times. All new infections need to be reported very quickly for the relevant bodies to put into place the right measures.

Stay Hydrated

Always make sure you are well hydrated, while you wait for medical attention. You should note, for now there is no vaccine that can contain the Ebola epidemic. The goal of all available treatments is to address the various symptoms, so as to make sure the patients are comfortable. You can use sports drinks or IV-drip for the rehydration purpose.

Control your blood pressure

A patient can easily be destabilized by rising blood pressure. However, If you experience a drop in blood pressure, then you might have been infected by a virus. It is the reason you should carefully monitor your blood pressure.

Ebola patients experience difficulty in breathing: that is why you would need an oxygen-rich environment. It will reduce the experience of chest pains, which is a common occurrence among infected people. Report any breathing difficulties to your nurses immediately.

Ensure that all symptoms are addressed as soon as possible:

Communicate openly with hospital staff in case of any discomfort. Inform them if you are experiencing a problem. For instance, if you are experiencing any infection, they can administer an antibiotic. It is important to be honest when you are explaining where you are experiencing pain.

Rest:

In case you acquire the virus, it is best to keep your body hydrated and allow yourself to rest. In nearly half of all the reported cases, the diseases are said to be fatal. Patients who have a good health, and healthy immune system are more likely to pull through. All they need is swift medical attention and other recovery treatments.

Update your knowledge on the available treatment options:

Stay abreast of all the available vaccines and treatments. As of yet, researchers haven't tested any of the potential vaccines on human beings. However, they are putting serious efforts in the development of an effective vaccine. The CDC website is the right place for you to check what the most recent treatments are.

A complete recovery from Ebola disease depends on the quality of healthcare services. The patient's immune system also plays a great role. People who recover from Ebola are known to develop antibodies that can last for up to ten years. In some cases, they last longer. In other cases, people who have recovered from Ebola develop other complications such as vision and joint problems.

Preliminary steps in controlling Ebola Virus

Researchers have found out that some cancer drugs may be capable of containing the spread of the Ebola virus. The Science Translation Medicine journal recently published a study on the effect of some leukemia drugs on Ebola patients. These drugs are imatinib and nilotinib and are sold by Novartis under the Gleevec and Tasigna brand names. These are two examples of tyrosine kinase inhibitors. It is an essential enzyme in facilitating the replication of Ebola virus as it makes it possible for the virus to spread throughout the body. The enzyme is responsible for transporting the phosphates into amino acids (that are a primary part of protein structure) and for protein function and shape.

These two drugs are effective in stopping the tumors associated with cancer. The prevent kinase from finalizing the process of cell reproduction. They prevent the reproduction of any hostile cells, leading to cell death. The name of this process is apoptosis. It is what ultimately stops the growth of tumors. Apparently, these drugs have affect the Ebola virus profoundly and prevent it from spreading quickly in the host's body.

A virus is a parasite, and that means that it requires a host cell in order to carry out the replication process. Otherwise, it will not be able to reproduce its genes. When the vital protein VP40 can no longer release the viral particles, the virus is unable to spread throughout the body. It means that the Ebola virus is limited to the host cells, and the body's immune system gets enough time to control the infection.

The First Case of Ebola

The Ebola hemorrhagic fever was first reported in the Republic of Zaire. This country has now changed its name to the Democratic Republic of Congo. The date was 28th August, 1976 when a middle-aged man complained of high fever at the Yambuku Catholic Mission in the northern part of Zaire. As usual the man was treated for malaria and then released. The nurses gave him an injection of chloroquine, which was the standard medication at that time. It proved to be useful at that point. After a period of three days, the fever returned with additional symptoms, one of them being gastrointestinal bleeding. The patient died while undergoing treatment.

Shortly afterwards, the Yambuku Catholic Mission closed down because 11 out of its 17 medical staff had died of the same symptoms like those of a man who complained of high fever earlier on. Subsequently, the disease reached 55 villages in the hospital neighborhood. Out of the 318 people who contracted the virus, 280 died.

Research, carried out later, indicated that the Yambuku Catholic Mission acted as a dissemination center for the Ebola virus. During this time, it was common for nurses to reuse syringes having just washed them in warm water. Healthcare professionals at the hospital often had to work with merely five syringes and needles for all patients. In some cases, the needles were boiled for reuse on the following day. The sanitary conditions were apparently allowing the Ebola virus to spread among the patients unchecked.

The Zaire outbreak of Ebola happened mainly due to the weak sterilization procedures at the hospital. Family members and relatives were infected by coming into close contact with patients.

The Zaire case was just the beginning of a series of other outbreaks in the African continent. Since, cases of Ebola have occurred in other countries such as Cote D'Ivoire, Uganda, Sudan, Nigeria, and Liberia among other countries.

In overall, over 1,850 cases of Ebola infections have been reported. Out of these known cases, 1200 people have died. Generally, the outbreaks tend to have high fatality rates.

Progress Vaccine Development

In December, 2011 researchers informed the public of the stage of development of new trial vaccines to counter the Ebola epidemic. These proved to be successful in protecting mice from infection, and the Proceedings of National Academy of Sciences journal reported breakthroughs in the development of the vaccine. The lead investigator was Charles Arntzen of the Arizona State University. The researcher determined that over 80 percent of the mice that received the four vaccinations over a period of two months survived after being infected by the Ebola virus.

The effectiveness of existing Ebola vaccines deteriorates over time. It is because the viral particles in such vaccines are damaged due to prolonged storage time. However, health workers claim the new vaccines contain an artificial version of the real Ebola virus, which allows them to vaccine remain viable having endured long storage. It makes it possible to create huge stockpiles of the essential vaccines, which governments can use to handle future Ebola outbreaks.

Complications

The Ebola virus proves to be deadly for a large number of people, who acquire it. With time, the illness leads to a coma, multiple organ failure, jaundice, shock, seizures, severe bleeding and delirium. The Ebola virus disease is exceedingly dangerous, as it destabilizes the immune system. Scientists are perplexed because some people recover from the virus while others do not.

The recovery process is very slow. It can take a lot of time for patients to regain their strength and weight, often several months. Due to the disease, people experience weakness, hair loss, liver inflation and sensory changes.

Quarantine

Quarantine is used to restrict and separate the movement of persons. The term means 'forced isolation'. It is an effective way to prevent any infectious disease from spreading. For example, in affected by outbreaks of the Ebola virus countries, schools and other public institutions are closed as an emergency measure. Keep in mind that US law allows officials to quarantine people who are infected by Ebola.

Chapter 7

When You Should Consider Leaving a Community Infected By Ebola

Living in areas, threatened by an Ebola outbreak, is quite a dangerous place so you should think about moving to a safer town. Since you have to move, you should ask yourself the following questions: "How safe is the new place I plan to move to?", "What will be the cost?", "If I acquire the virus while travelling, will I have access to medication?" In the case, all your answers are positive; you should move to a new location. Once you have made up your mind to travel, do not forget to carry personal protective equipment.

Ebola virus and its lifecycle

Human-to-human transmission takes place through direct contact with the bio fluids (this would include blood or any liquids in one's body) of anyone infected. Health workers should embalm an infected body, and any objects, touched by Ebola victims would need to be destroyed or sterilized thoroughly. It is quite important to remember when it comes to needles and syringes. All types of body fluids are known to be a major vehicle of transmission of the Ebola virus. Some of the most common fluids that you should not come into contact are tears, saliva, feces, vomit, sweat, urine, breast milk and semen. Usually, the virus enters the human body using various entry points such as the mouth, eyes, cuts, open wounds and abrasions.

Transmission from animals to humans occurs through the consumption of the meat of infected animals. It is extremely dangerous for people to consume apes and fruit bats. Healthcare organizations encourage all countries to support medical systems that are fully capable of following proper medical isolation procedures. In some cases, this is even a required measure.

Those infected with the Ebola virus cannot spread the disease widely because they are unable to travel far during the infectious stages. Researchers have always ruled out air as a medium for the transmission of the disease. It means that passengers who are sitting far from Ebola patients during air flights won't contract the virus. Traditional burial rituals are highly prohibited because bodies can still transmit the disease. A large number of Ebola infections in Guinea during the recent outbreak happened through unprotected contact with the deceased's bodies during burials. It is also vital to keep in mind that a male survivor's semen can remain infectious for seven weeks after the patient's recovery.

It is not very clear how the 2014 Ebola outbreak started. But people believe that the initial infection involved a human contact with animal body fluids.

Conclusion

Ebola is an extremely dangerous, rapidly spreading virus disease and poses a worldwide threat. For now, the largest epidemic has followed the outbreak in West African countries.

To ensure your protection from contracting the disease, you should follow the steps closely, outlined in this book. The different chapters clearly elaborate on all the issues, pertaining to Ebola.

The most recent, and deadliest outbreak of this deadly virus has stirred up international authorities and health institutions to act together to fight this common enemy to human health. Ebola is no match for one individual or a country, but requires our combined efforts to prevent it from becoming a global pandemic.

In any case, people should be better prepared for the threat of the Ebola virus. Being well informed is essential to protecting yourself and people around you, and this book offers all the necessary information on the subject.

Other Books By Ron Johnson

Prepper's Pantry

In the event of an emergency having an adequate supply of food could mean the difference between life and death! Are you prepared for any disaster that is about to happen? Do you already have emergency supplies? Is it enough to sustain you and your family's life for an extended period, when help from others would be close to impossible? Have you discussed and implemented the emergency plans with your family?

Fighting for your survival during times of disaster is not about luck, it's about the right knowledge that will help you pull through it. It is all about saving you and your family's life, with the tips provided in this book. Guess what? YOU CAN MAKE IT HAPPEN by reading and following all the guidelines laid out in this book.

RV Living For Beginners

Are You Fed Up Of Working The 9-5 To Pay The Mortgage Or Rent Plus The Bills And Considering Leaving It All Behind And Hitting The Road?

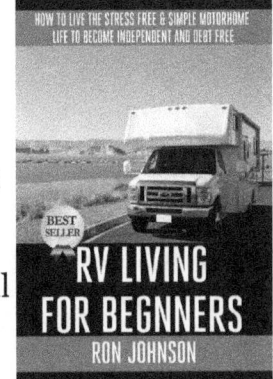

When you want to change your lifestyle entirely, you need to have enough motivation but you also need to have knowledge about the lifestyle that you are adopting. Many people who want to live in an RV full-time fail to find a balance in their lives which make that living pleasurable, while others can live the dream and learn to compromise on comforts for the sake of freedom. They wake up in the mornings to feel that they have breathed fresh air. They see different scenery every morning if they so wish. What you need to know before joining them is whether you're cut out for the lifestyle and what differences there are between living in a conventional home and living in an RV. This book bridges that gap in your knowledge, and although you may choose to save a fortune by staying at home, you may also choose the lesser travelled road and discover the benefits of living in an RV.

Both lifestyles, either in an RV or a home, have their pros and cons. Many who choose the RV lifestyle find that adapting their lives comes naturally. It takes a unique and free spirited person to compromise on the luxuries of home living in favor of the adventurous lifestyle offered by RV living, though many do. Once you weigh the pros and cons, you can make the choice wisely, and that's what this book is all about. The book will appeal to the free spirited who seek something more than merely surviving month to month oppressed by bills, mortgage payments and housing taxes.

Both have benefits, though those who live the life they choose, rather than the life chosen for them by responsibility, find that RV life tests their personal boundaries and skills freeing up their lives to live beyond the grid. Journey with us and learn if living in an RV will suit you, and be prepared for the journey of your life.

www.ingramcontent.com/pod-product-compliance
Lightning Source LLC
Chambersburg PA
CBHW070518290526
45790CB00003B/1253